Dog Nutrition for Beginners 2024

The Complete Guide to Feeding Your Pet for
Optimal Health and Longevity

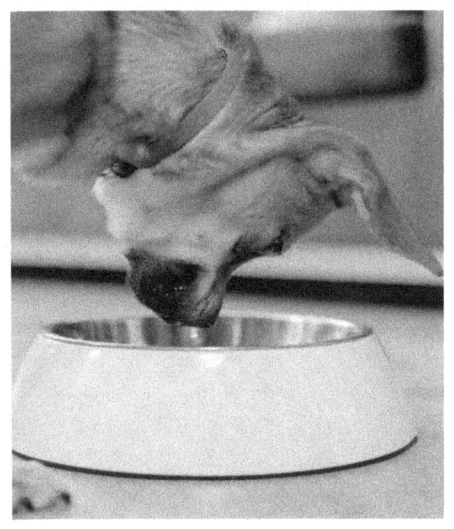

Silas Bardwell

For the lovers of Man's best friends

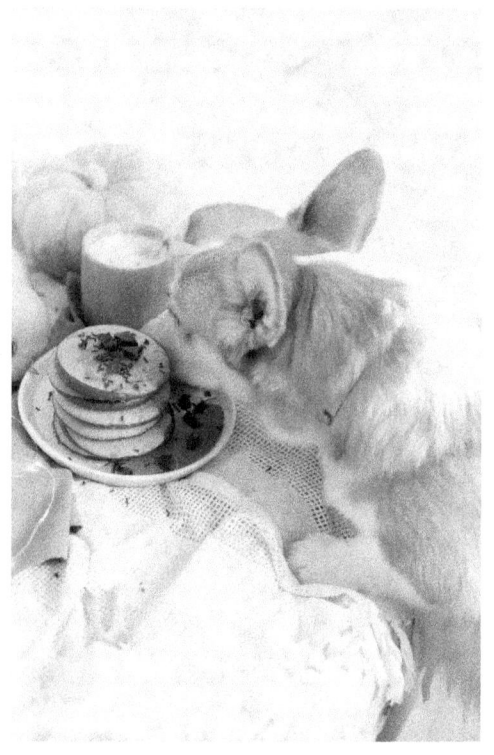

Copyright © 2024 by Silas Bardwell

TABLE OF CONTENTS

Introduction

When I first got my dog, Max, I was determined to provide him the best care possible, including adequate nourishment. I conducted significant study and talked with vets to determine Max's specific nutritional requirements depending on his breed and age. I learned about the nutrients that dogs require and how to provide him with a balanced diet to maintain his general health and well-being.

I decided to feed Max a mix of high-quality commercial dog food and homemade meals customized to his specific needs. I carefully read and analysed dog food labels to find solutions that delivered the essential nutrition while avoiding extraneous fillers and additives. I changed Max's food as he grew older to fit his changing activity level and metabolism, ensuring he received the best nutrients for his age.

Max has maintained a healthy weight, a lustrous coat, and unlimited vitality as a result of this strategy. He has also avoided the normal health problems connected with inadequate eating and thrived into his elderly years. I have witnessed personally the influence of correct nutrition on Max's health and longevity, and I am determined to providing him with the greatest food possible for the remainder of his life. This experience has reaffirmed my conviction that knowing canine nutrition and its role in ensuring our cherished animals live robust and fulfilled lives is critical.

The importance of proper nutrition for dogs

Proper nutrition is critical for dogs' general health and well-being. Dogs, like humans, require a well-balanced diet rich in nutrients to support their growth, development, and overall health. Proper nutrition is critical for dogs' longevity, energy levels, and resistance to common health conditions.

In the case of Max, the decision to feed him a mix of high-quality commercial dog food and handmade meals tailored to his specific needs was critical to ensuring he received the best nutrition for his breed and age. Max's owner was able to guarantee that he received a balanced diet that supported his overall health by carefully reading dog food labels and picking products that supplied important nutrients without needless fillers or additives.

Puppy nutrition is very important since they need a diet that supports their rapid growth and development. Puppies require a meal high in protein, vitamins, and minerals to help maintain their growing muscles, bones, and organs. Puppy growth may be stunted, immune systems impaired, and other health issues may occur if sufficient nutrition is not provided during this vital stage of development.

Dogs' nutritional demands fluctuate as they age, and it is vital to adapt their food to meet their increasing activity level and metabolism. Senior dogs may require a diet that is reduced in calories while still providing the nutrients their bodies require as they age. Senior dogs who do not receive sufficient nourishment may be more prone to obesity, joint difficulties, and other age-related health issues.

The importance of knowing dog nutrition is demonstrated by the influence of good diet on Max's health and longevity. Giving dogs a balanced diet that fulfils their individual nutritional demands will help them avoid common health problems associated with inadequate nutrition, such as obesity, digestive disorders, and skin problems. It can also help them with their energy levels, coat health, and immune function.

The significance of good nourishment for dogs cannot be overstated. Understanding your dog's individual dietary needs based on breed, age, and activity level is critical to delivering the best care possible. We can support dogs' overall health and well-being and help them live vibrant and meaningful lives by ensuring that they receive a balanced diet that provides important nutrients without needless fillers or additions.

How good nutrition contributes to optimal health and longevity

Good nutrition is vital for dogs' general health and longevity. Max, my beloved dog, is a wonderful illustration of how good nutrition can help you live a longer and healthier life. I was able to provide Max with the best nutrition for his breed and age by feeding him a combination of high-quality commercial dog food and homemade meals suited to his specific needs.

First and foremost, proper diet is critical for a dog's growth and development. When Max was a puppy, I made careful to provide him a high-protein, vitamin-and-mineral-rich food to encourage his quick growth and development. This ensured appropriate development of his muscles, bones, and organs, laying the groundwork for a healthy and robust adult dog.

I changed Max's food as he grew older to meet his growing activity level and metabolism. This is significant because the nutritional requirements of dogs alter as they mature. Senior dogs may require a diet that is reduced in calories while still providing the nutrients their bodies require as they age. I was able to support Max's general health and well-being as he approached his golden years by providing him with a diet customized to his specific needs as a senior dog.

Proper nutrition is also important for a dog's energy levels, coat quality, and immunological function. I was able to feed Max with a balanced diet that supported his general health by carefully reading dog food labels and picking products that supplied important nutrients without needless fillers or additives. As a result, his overall energy levels and coat health improved, keeping him lively and active throughout his life.

Furthermore, excellent nutrition can help prevent common health problems associated with poor nutrition, such as obesity, digestive disorders, and skin problems. I was able to assist avert these health issues and promote Max's overall well-being by feeding him with a balanced meal that addressed his individual nutritional demands.

Finally, excellent diet is critical for a dog's overall health and lifespan. You can provide your dog with the best possible care if you understand their individual dietary needs depending on their breed, age, and activity level.

Max's health and longevity are testaments to the importance of proper nutrition for dogs, and we can support their overall health and well-being by ensuring that they receive a balanced diet that provides essential nutrients without unnecessary fillers or additives, allowing them to live vibrant and fulfilling lives.

Chapter 1: Understanding Your Dog's Nutritional Needs

Understanding your dog's nutritional requirements is critical to their general health and lifespan. Dogs, like humans, require a well-balanced diet rich in critical nutrients to support their growth, development, and overall health. As a dog owner, I've learnt the value of understanding my dog's unique nutritional requirements and adjusting their food to ensure they get the best nutrition for their breed and age.

Max, my beloved dog, is a wonderful illustration of how good nutrition can help you live a longer and healthier life. I was able to establish his exact nutritional needs by thoroughly evaluating his breed, age, and activity level, and providing him with a combination of high-quality commercial dog food and cooked meals suited to his individual needs. This enabled me to guarantee that Max received a well-balanced diet rich in important nutrients and free of needless fillers and additives, so maintaining his overall health and well-being throughout his life.

We will look at how understanding your dog's nutritional needs can help with their growth, development, energy levels, coat health, and immunological function. You may help prevent common health issues connected with poor nutrition and promote your dog's general health and longevity by understanding and satisfying his or her individual dietary needs.

Dogs, like humans, require a range of critical nutrients to maintain good health and well-being. Protein, carbs, lipids, vitamins, and minerals are among the nutrients that are essential for their growth, development, energy levels, coat health, and immune function.

The Essential Nutrients for Dogs

Protein is a vital food for dogs since it serves as the foundation for muscle development and repair. It is also essential for maintaining a healthy immune system and encouraging general growth and development. High-quality protein sources, such as chicken, beef, fish, and eggs, are essential components of a dog's diet to ensure they get the amino acids they need for maximum health.

Carbohydrates give dogs energy and fiber to help with digestion. While dogs do not require as many carbohydrates as people, nutritious grains, fruits, and vegetables can help boost their energy levels and overall well-being.

Fats are an important nutrient for dogs because they provide a concentrated source of energy and aid in the absorption of fat-soluble vitamins. Omega-3 and Omega-6 fatty acids are very crucial for skin and coat health, brain function, and inflammation reduction.

Vitamins and minerals are required for many biological activities in dogs. Vitamin A, for example, is essential for vision and immunological function, while Vitamin D promotes bone health and Vitamin E functions as an antioxidant to protect cells from damage. Calcium, phosphorus, and potassium are minerals that are necessary for bone health, muscle function, and overall well-being.

Water, in addition to these necessary elements, is essential for a dog's overall health. Adequate hydration is required for appropriate digestion, body temperature regulation, and overall bodily processes.

Understanding your dog's particular dietary requirements is critical for ensuring they get the right combination of these key nutrients. When determining the optimum food for your dog, consider factors such as breed, age, size, activity level, and any underlying health concerns. You can assist promote their general health and longevity by providing a balanced diet that fulfills their individual nutritional demands, while also reducing common health conditions associated with poor nutrition.

Understanding the essential nutrients for dogs and adapting their food to their specific needs is critical for maintaining their growth, development, energy levels, coat health, and immune function. You can help preserve your dog's optimal health and longevity by giving a balanced diet that includes high-quality amounts of protein, carbs, fats, vitamins, minerals, and appropriate hydration.

How to determine your dog's specific nutritional requirements

Determining your dog's individual nutritional needs entails taking into account a number of elements that can influence their food requirements. Breed, age, size, activity level, and any underlying health issues are among these considerations. Taking these elements into consideration allows you to design your dog's food to fulfil their particular nutritional demands while also supporting their overall health and well-being.

The nutritional requirements of different dog breeds vary. Large breeds, for example, may require a diet that promotes healthy bone growth and joint health, whereas small breeds may require a higher-calorie diet to sustain their fast metabolism. Understanding your dog's breed's individual demands will help you choose the proper sort and amount of food for them.

Puppies, adult dogs, and senior dogs have distinct nutritional requirements. Puppies need a diet that promotes quick growth and development, but senior dogs may benefit from a diet that promotes joint health and cognitive function. Understanding your dog's life stage will assist you in selecting a food that matches their individual demands.

Size: Your dog's nutritional requirements may be influenced by their size. Large breeds may require a diet that promotes good bone growth, whereas small breeds may require a higher-calorie diet to sustain their quick metabolism. Understanding your dog's size might assist you in selecting the appropriate type and amount of food for them.

Activity Level: Active dogs may require a higher calorie diet to meet their energy needs, whereas less active dogs may benefit from a reduced calorie diet to avoid weight gain. Understanding your dog's activity level might assist you in selecting a food that suits their individual requirements.

Underlying Health disorders: Dogs with underlying health disorders, such as allergies, digestive issues, or kidney illness, may require a customized diet to meet their unique requirements. Consult your veterinarian to decide the appropriate diet for your dog depending on their specific health concerns.

I talked with my veterinarian to assess Max's nutritional requirements. They were able to make tailored suggestions for Max based on his breed, age, size, activity level, and overall health. They suggested a high-quality dog food with the proper combination of protein, carbohydrates, fats, vitamins, and minerals to meet Max's unique requirements. They also advised Max on portion control and feeding frequency to ensure he was getting the right quantity of food for his size and activity level.

I was able to assess Max's unique nutritional needs and give him with a balanced diet that supported his overall health and well-being by taking these elements into account and consulting with a veterinarian. Regular veterinarian visits enabled me to make changes to Max's food as he aged and his demands changed, ensuring that he obtained the nutrients he required for optimal health and longevity.

Factors to consider when choosing the right diet for your dog

There are several key elements to consider when selecting the correct food for your dog in order to satisfy their individual nutritional needs. Breed, age, size, activity level, and any underlying health issues are among these considerations.

The breed of your dog has a huge impact on their nutritional requirements. distinct breeds have distinct nutritional requirements, and understanding these variances will assist you in selecting the correct sort and amount of food for your dog. Large breeds, for example, may require a diet that promotes healthy bone growth and joint health, whereas small breeds may require a higher-calorie diet to sustain their fast metabolism.

Another important issue to consider when assessing your dog's nutritional requirements is age. Puppies, adult dogs, and senior dogs all have distinct nutritional needs. Puppies need a diet that promotes quick growth and development, but senior dogs may benefit from a diet that promotes joint health and cognitive function.

When selecting a diet for your dog, you need also consider their size. Large breeds may require a diet that promotes good bone growth, whereas small breeds may require a higher-calorie diet to sustain their quick metabolism.

Another aspect that can influence your dog's dietary demands is their amount of activity. Active dogs may require a higher-calorie diet to meet their energy requirements, whilst less active dogs may benefit from a lower-calorie diet to avoid weight gain.

Finally, any underlying health concerns your dog may have should be considered when selecting a diet. Dogs suffering from allergies, digestive difficulties, or kidney illness may require a particular diet to meet their individual requirements. Consult your veterinarian to decide the appropriate diet for your dog depending on their specific health concerns.

Selecting the best diet for your dog entails taking into account a number of aspects that can influence their dietary requirements. You may adapt your dog's diet to fit their particular nutritional needs and promote their general health and well-being by considering their breed, age, size, activity level, and any underlying health concerns. A veterinarian can provide individualized advice and guidance on portion control and feeding frequency to ensure that your dog is getting the right quantity of food for their size and activity level. By taking these variables into consideration and getting professional advice, you can give your dog with a balanced diet that meets their individual demands while also promoting optimal health and longevity.

Chapter 2: Commercial Dog Food vs. Homemade Dog Food

As pet owners, we all want what is best for our pets, especially when it comes to nutrition. What we feed our pets is one of the most crucial decisions we can make for them. With so many alternatives, deciding between commercial dog food and homemade dog food might be difficult. Both have advantages and downsides, and it is critical to thoroughly examine these factors before making a decision.

Commercial dog food is convenient and widely available, with a variety of options to meet a variety of dietary needs and tastes. It is designed to suit the nutritional needs of dogs and frequently includes extra vitamins and minerals to ensure a balanced diet. Homemade dog food, on the other hand, gives pet owners complete control over the ingredients and quality of the food they serve their pets. It may be customized to match individual dietary requirements and is an excellent choice for dogs with allergies or sensitivities.

We will compare commercial dog food to homemade dog food, including the nutritional content, cost, convenience, and potential health benefits and hazards connected with each alternative. Pet owners can make an informed decision about what sort of food is best for their cherished canine friends by considering these considerations. Finally, while evaluating their diet, we should prioritize our dogs' health and well-being, and understanding the advantages and downsides of both commercial and homemade dog food is critical in making the appropriate choice.

The pros and cons of commercial dog food

Commercial dog food has a number of benefits that make it a popular choice among pet owners. One of the most significant advantages of commercial dog food is its ease of use. It is widely available in pet stores, grocery stores, and online, making it simple for pet owners to buy and store. Commercial dog food is also available in a variety of forms, including dry kibble, canned food, and semi-moist food, as well as formulae tailored to different life stages, breeds, and nutritional requirements. This diversity makes it simple for pet owners to pick a food that suits their dog's nutritional needs.

Another benefit of commercial dog food is that it is designed to suit the nutritional requirements of dogs. Most commercial dog feeds are designed with the help of veterinary nutritionists and are rigorously tested to guarantee that they provide a balanced diet for dogs. They frequently include additional vitamins, minerals, and other critical ingredients to promote general health and well-being. Furthermore, many commercial dog diets are formulated to target specific health conditions, such as weight management, joint health, and digestive disorders.

Despite these benefits, commercial dog food has certain disadvantages. One of the most serious issues with commercial dog food is the quality of the ingredients. Some commercial dog diets may contain fillers, byproducts, artificial additives, and preservatives that are not appropriate for a dog's diet. Pet owners must carefully study the ingredient list and select high-quality commercial dog diets that emphasize real meat, healthy grains, and natural additives.

When it comes to commercial dog food, price is another element to consider. While there are low-cost options, some high-quality commercial dog foods can be costly, especially for larger breeds or dogs with special nutritional requirements. Furthermore, the cost of commercial dog food can quickly add up, especially for pet owners who have many dogs.

Finally, commercial dog food provides convenience and a variety of options for meeting the nutritional needs of dogs. However, while selecting a commercial dog food for their pets, pet owners should consider the quality of the components as well as the price. It is critical to conduct research and select a high-quality commercial dog food that contains key nutrients and promotes dogs' general health and well-being.

How to make balanced and nutritious homemade dog food

Making balanced and nutritious homemade dog food can be a terrific alternative to commercial dog food, especially for pet owners worried about ingredient quality and wanting more control over their dog's nutrition. Pet owners can guarantee that their homemade dog food contains all of the important nutrients their canines require by following a few simple instructions.

To identify the exact nutritional needs of the dog, the first step in preparing homemade dog food is to confer with a veterinarian or veterinary nutritionist. This will assist pet owners in understanding the proper protein, carbohydrate, fat, vitamin, and mineral balance that should be included in homemade dog food.

After determining the nutritional requirements, pet owners may begin picking high-quality ingredients for their homemade dog food. Lean meats like chicken, turkey, beef, and fish are high in protein and should be the main element in homemade dog food. It is critical to fully prepare the meat before incorporating it in the dog's food to eradicate any hazardous microorganisms.

Homemade dog food should include healthful carbs such as brown rice, sweet potatoes, and quinoa in addition to meat. These components provide energy and fiber to the digestive system of the dog. Carrots, peas, apples, and blueberries are examples of fruits and vegetables that can be added to give necessary vitamins, minerals, and antioxidants.

Pet owners should incorporate a source of healthy fats such as fish oil or flaxseed oil in their homemade dog food to ensure that it is well-balanced. These fats are necessary for a healthy coat and skin, as well as for overall health and well-being.

Certain items, including as onions, garlic, grapes, raisins, and chocolate, should be avoided while creating homemade dog food since they can be poisonous to dogs. Furthermore, bones should never be included in homemade dog food because they might splinter and harm the dog's digestive tract.

After selecting all of the ingredients, pet owners can produce homemade dog food by heating the meat and carbohydrates separately and then combining them in proper portions. It is critical to manage portion sizes to ensure that the dog is getting enough nutrients for their size and activity level.

Overall, producing balanced and healthy homemade dog food necessitates careful consideration of the dog's individual nutritional requirements as well as the use of high-quality components. While it may take more time and work than purchasing commercial dog food, homemade dog food can give pet owners piece of mind knowing exactly what their pets are eating and can contribute to their pets' general health and well-being.

Tips for ensuring your homemade dog food meets your dog's nutritional needs

Adapting your dog's food to their activity level is a crucial part of ensuring that they get the right balance of nutrients to support their general health and well-being. Dogs, like humans, have variable levels of activity and energy consumption, and their diet should be tailored to fit their particular requirements. Here are some suggestions for modifying your dog's food based on their level of activity:

1. measure Your Dog's Activity Level: The first step in modifying your dog's diet is to measure their activity level. Dogs that are very active, such as working dogs, agility dogs, or those that indulge in regular exercise, will have

higher energy requirements compared to sedentary or less active dogs.

2. contact with a Veterinarian: Before making any changes to your dog's diet, it is vital to contact with a veterinarian or veterinary nutritionist to identify the right alterations based on your dog's individual needs. They may provide recommendations on the appropriate balance of protein, carbs, fats, vitamins, and minerals that should be included in your dog's diet based on their activity level.

3. Increase Protein consumption: For highly active dogs, increasing the protein consumption in their food can assist support their muscular development and repair. Lean meats like chicken, turkey, steak, and fish are high in protein and should be included in larger amounts for energetic dogs.

4. Adjust Carbohydrate Intake: Because carbs offer energy for your dog's activities, the amount of healthy carbohydrates in their diet should be adjusted dependent on their activity level. Active dogs may require more carbohydrates, such as brown rice, sweet potatoes, and quinoa, to meet their energy requirements.

5. Monitor Portion Sizes: It is critical to monitor portion sizes to ensure that your dog is getting enough nutrients for their size and activity level. Active dogs may require bigger portion sizes to meet their energy needs, whilst less active dogs may require fewer portion sizes to avoid weight gain.

6. Consider Nutrient Supplements: To maintain their overall health and well-being, extremely active dogs may benefit from nutrient supplements such as fish oil or multivitamins. These supplements can assist them address nutritional deficiencies in their diet while also supporting their increased energy expenditure.

7. Hydration: Regardless of activity level, it is critical that your dog always has access to fresh, clean water. Active dogs may need extra water to be hydrated, particularly during periods of high physical activity. You can ensure that your dog receives the proper balance of nutrients to support their energy needs, muscle development, and overall health by modifying their food based on their activity level. It is critical to consult with a veterinarian or veterinary nutritionist in order to make informed decisions about your dog's diet and guarantee that they flourish based on their unique activity level.

Tips for ensuring your homemade dog food meets your dog's nutritional needs

When making homemade dog food, make sure it matches your dog's nutritional needs, particularly in proportion to their activity level. Here are some pointers to follow to ensure that your homemade dog food contains the proper nutrient balance to support your dog's general health and well-being:

1. speak with a Veterinarian: Before making homemade dog food, speak with a veterinarian or veterinary nutritionist to verify the proper nutrient balance depending on your dog's individual needs. They can advise you on the best protein, carbohydrate, fat, vitamin, and mineral mix for your dog's homemade diet according on their activity level.

2. Determine Your Dog's Activity Level: Just as with conventional dog food, it is critical to determine your dog's activity level when making homemade dog food. Highly active dogs have increased energy needs and may require a diet rich in protein and healthy carbs to meet those needs.

3. High-Quality Protein Sources: When making homemade dog food, use high-quality protein sources including lean

meats (chicken, turkey, cattle, fish), eggs, and lentils. These protein sources are critical for muscle building and repair, particularly in highly active dogs.

4. Carbohydrate Balance: Because carbs give energy for your dog's activity, it's critical to include healthy carbohydrates in their homemade diet, such as brown rice, sweet potatoes, quinoa, and veggies. Adjust the carbohydrate amount based on your dog's activity level to ensure they have enough energy to thrive.

5. Healthy Fats: Including healthy fats in your dog's homemade diet, such as fish oil, coconut oil, and olive oil, can give important fatty acids to promote their general health and well-being. Healthy fats can also supply additional energy to sustain extremely active dogs' higher energy expenditure.

6. Monitor Portion Sizes: When making homemade dog food, it's critical to keep track of portion sizes to ensure that your dog gets the correct amount of nutrients for his or her size and activity level. To meet their energy needs without gaining weight, adjust meal sizes based on their activity level.

7. Consider Nutrient Supplements: Depending on your dog's unique needs and activity level, nutrient supplements such as fish oil or multivitamins may be beneficial in filling any nutritional gaps in their homemade diet.

You may verify that your homemade dog food fits your dog's nutritional demands based on their activity level by following these suggestions and consulting with a veterinarian or veterinary nutritionist. A well-balanced, nutrient-dense homemade meal can help your dog's energy levels, muscle development, and overall wellness.

Chapter 3: Reading Dog Food Labels

Every pet owner should be able to read dog food labels. We endeavor to give the greatest nutrition for our animal buddies as responsible guardians. With so many alternatives on the market, reading the information on dog food labels may be daunting and perplexing. Understanding these labels is critical to ensure that our dogs are fed a nutritious and well-balanced diet.

Dog food labels offer vital information regarding the product's ingredients, nutritional composition, and feeding requirements. Pet owners can make informed selections about which dog food is best for their canine companions by carefully inspecting these labels. The ingredients list is very important because it gives information about the food's quality and composition. Choosing a dog food that has high-quality protein sources, such as real meat, should be a top consideration.

Understanding the nutritional content is also important for satisfying our pets' individual dietary needs. Dog food labels often include information regarding the product's protein, fat, and carbohydrate content. It is important to remember that different breeds and life phases may necessitate different nutrient ratios, so contact with a veterinarian to discover the best nutritional profile for your dog.

Reading dog food labels can also assist in identifying potential allergens or components that may be hazardous to our pets. Certain substances, such as grains or certain proteins, may cause sensitivities or allergies in some dogs. Pet owners can avoid purchasing goods that may cause unpleasant responses in their dogs by carefully reading the labels.

Finally, reading dog food labels is an important activity for pet owners who value their dogs' health and well-being. We can make informed judgments regarding the best dog food options for our furry companions by researching the ingredients, nutritional content, and potential allergens.

Understanding the ingredients list

Understanding the ingredients list is critical when it comes to making informed food choices. In today's environment, where processed and packaged foods predominate, it's critical to be cognizant of what we put into our bodies. The components list gives useful information about a product's makeup, including any potential allergens or dangerous compounds.

First and foremost, knowing the contents list allows us to identify any potential allergens in a product. This information is critical for those who have food allergies or intolerances to maintain their safety and well-being. Reading the ingredients list attentively can quickly reveal whether a product contains common allergens such as peanuts, gluten, or dairy. This knowledge enables people to make informed decisions about whether a product is appropriate for their nutritional needs.

Additionally, the components list assists us in identifying any possibly dangerous compounds that may be present in a product. Many processed meals contain artificial additives, preservatives, and taste enhancers, all of which can be harmful to human health. We can avoid products that contain these compounds if we are familiar with them and understand their possible hazards. Some studies, for example, have connected specific food colorings to hyperactivity in youngsters, while others have suggested that artificial sweeteners may be harmful to metabolism. We can deliberately avoid such chemicals by reviewing the ingredients list and prioritizing better options.

Furthermore, comprehending the ingredients list allows us to analyze a product's nutritional value. Typically, the list begins with the most plentiful element and progresses in declining order. This indicates that if the first few ingredients of a product include harmful fats, refined sugars, or highly processed grains, it might not be the ideal choice for a balanced diet. If, on the other hand, entire foods such as fruits, vegetables, or whole grains are listed first, it implies a better composition. Understanding the components list allows us to make decisions that are in line with our dietary goals and overall well-being.

Finally, knowing the ingredients fosters transparency in the food market. It enables customers to hold firms accountable for the ingredients they use in their goods. Individuals can make better informed purchasing selections when they are aware of the ingredients they should avoid or prioritize. This rising demand for healthier, more transparent food options may prompt corporations to enhance their formulas and offer products that are more in line with consumer expectations.

Comprehending the ingredients list is critical for making informed food decisions. It aids in the identification of potential allergies, the avoidance of dangerous compounds, the assessment of nutritional value, and the promotion of transparency in the food sector. We can prioritize our health and well-being while contributing to a more conscious and responsible food culture by taking the time to read and understand the ingredients list.

Identifying high-quality dog food options

Finding high-quality dog food options is critical for our canine companions' health and well-being. Understanding the ingredients list is critical when it comes to making informed decisions about what we feed our dogs, just as it is with human food.

To begin, reading the ingredients list allows us to discover any potential allergens in a dog food product. Many dogs have food allergies or intolerances, and feeding them a diet containing their allergens can cause discomfort, digestive disorders, and even more serious health concerns. We can quickly detect if a dog food contains common allergens like chicken, beef, wheat, or soy by carefully inspecting the ingredients list. This knowledge enables us to select a dog food that is appropriate for our pet's individual nutritional demands and aids in the prevention of allergic reactions.

Understanding the ingredients list also assists us in identifying any possibly dangerous compounds that may be present in a dog food product. Many commercial dog diets, like processed human foods, contain artificial additives, preservatives, and fillers that can be harmful to our dogs' health. These additives can cause allergies, digestive disorders, and even long-term health problems including obesity or heart disease. We may avoid dog diets that include these additives and choose for products that value natural and healthful ingredients if we are familiar with them and recognize their possible consequences.

Furthermore, the ingredients list enables us to determine the nutritional content of a dog food product. A balanced diet that combines high-quality proteins, healthy fats, and necessary nutrients is required for dogs. We can confirm that the dog food we purchase contains real meat sources as the major ingredient, rather than fillers or by-products, by reviewing the ingredients list. We can also look for entire grains, fruits, and vegetables, which are high in vitamins and minerals. Avoiding dog diets that are high in carbs or artificial flavors and colors is also critical for our dogs' general health and vigor.

Finally, knowing the ingredients fosters transparency in the pet food market. It enables us to hold firms responsible for the quality of the ingredients used in their goods. When we know what to look for in high-quality dog food, we can make more informed shopping decisions and choose companies that prioritize our pets' health and well-being. Because of the rising need for transparent and healthy dog food options, companies may improve their formulations and offer goods that satisfy the expectations of responsible pet owners.

Finally, when it comes to finding high-quality dog food options, reading the ingredients list is critical. It aids in the identification of potential allergies, the avoidance of dangerous compounds, the assessment of nutritional value, and the promotion of openness in the pet food sector. We can prioritize the health and well-being of our beloved dogs while contributing to a more conscientious and ethical pet food culture by taking the time to read and comprehend the ingredients list.

How to avoid common pitfalls when choosing dog food

A dog's food should be adjusted based on their activity level to ensure their overall health and well-being. Dogs, like humans, have varied energy requirements based on their activity levels, and feeding them with the proper nutritional balance is critical for their maximum performance and general health.

There are several crucial elements to consider when adjusting a dog's food based on their activity level:

1. Determine the dog's level of activity: Begin by determining how active your dog is on a daily basis. Take into account their breed, age, size, and activity schedule. Working or sporting breeds, for example, will require more calories and nutrients than dogs who live a more sedentary lifestyle.

2. Consult with a veterinarian: Before making any big modifications to your dog's food, it is always best to

consult with a veterinarian. They can offer advice tailored to your dog's specific needs and assist in determining the right dietary modifications based on their activity level.

3. Changing portion sizes: After assessing your dog's activity level and consulting with a veterinarian, you can change their portion quantities as needed. Dogs who are more active will require greater portions to meet their energy requirements. Dogs with lower activity levels, on the other hand, may require lesser servings to avoid weight gain and maintain a healthy physical condition.

4. Choosing the proper food: Choosing the right dog food is critical for addressing your dog's nutritional needs. To meet the energy requirements of extremely active dogs, choose a dog food with a greater protein and fat content. Look for high-quality dog foods with actual meat as the main ingredient. Consider selections that include healthy carbohydrates for long-term energy and critical nutrients for general health.

5. Weight monitoring and adjustment as needed: Check your dog's weight and body condition on a regular basis to ensure they are maintaining a healthy weight. If your dog

starts gaining or losing weight, you may need to change their portion levels or move to a new type of dog food that better meets their needs.

6. Providing additional supplements as needed: Your veterinarian may offer additional supplements such as omega-3 fatty acids or joint support supplements based on your dog's individual needs and activity level. These can help maintain their overall health and address any specific issues about their level of activity.

Finally, modifying a dog's diet based on their activity level is critical for overall health and well-being. We can ensure that our dogs receive the appropriate balance of nutrients to support their energy requirements and promote optimal health by assessing their activity level, consulting with a veterinarian, adjusting portion sizes, choosing the right type of food, monitoring weight, and providing additional supplements as needed.

Chapter 4: Special Dietary Considerations for Dogs

Dietary considerations for dogs with certain health issues are critical to their overall health and well-being. Dogs, like humans, can acquire a variety of health issues that may necessitate dietary changes to manage their symptoms and support their general health.

When it comes to dogs who have special health challenges, such as obesity, diabetes, allergies, or gastrointestinal disorders, it is even more crucial to adjust their diet to match their specific needs. These illnesses frequently necessitate dietary changes to help manage symptoms, regulate weight, and enhance overall quality of life.

Dogs suffering from obesity, for example, may benefit from a weight control diet low in calories and fat. Diabetes in dogs may necessitate a diet low in carbohydrates and high in fiber to help regulate blood sugar levels. To avoid causing allergic reactions, dogs with allergies or food sensitivities may require a limited ingredient or hypoallergenic diet. Dogs suffering from gastrointestinal disorders may benefit from a food that is easily digestible and has nutrients that promote gut health.

It is critical to check with a veterinarian to determine the appropriate dietary plan for dogs with unique health conditions. They can advise on suitable dietary changes, recommend specialist dog meals or therapeutic diets, and monitor their progress to guarantee optimal results.

We can effectively manage their symptoms, improve their overall health, and increase their quality of life by taking these special dietary concerns for dogs with specific health conditions into account.

Nutrition for puppies and senior dogs

Nutrition for puppies and older dogs is extremely important when it comes to their overall health and well-being, particularly when it comes to specific health concerns. Puppies and older dogs, like dogs with other health issues, may require dietary changes to meet their specific demands.

Puppies have different nutritional needs than adult dogs. They are in a period of rapid growth and development, thus their diet should be specially designed to supply the nutrients required for optimal growth. Puppies' growing bodies necessitate increased doses of protein, fat, vitamins, and minerals. It is critical to give them with a balanced and comprehensive puppy diet to ensure they acquire all of the necessary nutrients they require.

Puppies may also have special health issues that necessitate nutritional changes. Some dogs, for example, may develop food allergies or sensitivities, necessitating a limited ingredient or hypoallergenic diet. It is critical to detect any potential allergies or sensitivities early on and make the appropriate dietary changes to avoid allergic reactions and boost general health.

Senior dogs, on the other hand, have different nutritional requirements than adult dogs and puppies. Dogs' metabolism decreases as they age, and they may become less active. This can result in weight gain as well as an increased risk of certain health disorders like obesity and joint difficulties. As a result, elderly dogs may benefit from a diet reduced in calories and fat content to help them maintain a healthy weight and maintain joint health.

Senior dogs may also have medical issues that necessitate nutritional changes. Many senior dogs, for example, suffer from age-related illnesses such as arthritis or kidney disease. These disorders may necessitate dietary changes to manage symptoms and support overall health. A senior dog diet may include elements that promote joint health or are easier to digest for dogs suffering from kidney disease.

Finally, diet for puppies and older dogs is critical in relation to their individual health concerns. Puppies require a balanced and comprehensive food to support their quick growth and development, but elderly dogs may benefit from a diet that helps them maintain a healthy weight while also meeting their special health needs. Consultation with a veterinarian is essential to ensure that the proper nutritional adjustments are made to meet the individual demands of puppies and elderly dogs, thereby encouraging their general health and well-being.

Dietary considerations for dogs with specific health conditions

Dietary considerations for dogs suffering from various medical disorders are critical to their overall health and well-being. Dogs with specific health concerns, such pups and senior dogs, may require dietary changes to suit their individual demands and effectively manage their health conditions.

Food allergies or sensitivities are a prevalent health problem in dogs. When dogs with food allergies consume particular substances, they may develop symptoms such as itching, gastrointestinal problems, or skin irritations. In such circumstances, a low-ingredient or hypoallergenic diet may be advised. These diets include fewer ingredients, making it easier to detect and remove potential allergies. They are frequently designed using innovative protein and carbohydrate sources that are less prone to cause allergic reactions. Dogs with food allergies can get relief from their symptoms and improve their overall health by consuming a diet free of allergic components.

Obesity is another health problem that may necessitate dietary changes. Obesity in dogs can cause a variety of health difficulties, including musculoskeletal problems, diabetes, and cardiovascular disease. A diet low in calories and fat content is usually recommended to manage weight and aid weight loss. These diets frequently contain more fiber to help dogs feel full while consuming less calories. Additionally, weight management diets may include components that promote joint health, such as glucosamine and chondroitin, to relieve joint stress caused by excess weight.

Dietary changes may also be required for dogs with kidney disease. Kidney disease impairs the kidneys' ability to filter waste products from the blood, causing toxins to build up in the body. For dogs with kidney disease, a low-phosphorus, high-quality protein diet is usually advised. These diets help to lessen the workload on the kidneys and the accumulation of waste products. They may also contain omega-3 fatty acids, antioxidants, and B vitamins, which can help with kidney function and overall health.

Finally, dogs with arthritis or joint disorders may benefit from a joint-healthy diet. These diets frequently include components like glucosamine, chondroitin, and omega-3 fatty acids, which aid in inflammation reduction and joint mobility. Furthermore, diets designed for dogs with joint difficulties may be lower in calories to minimize weight gain, which can exacerbate joint problems.

Finally, nutritional considerations for dogs suffering from certain health concerns are critical to their overall health and well-being. Whether it's food allergies, obesity, kidney illness, or joint pain, tailoring their diet to their specific needs can help them manage their health concerns more effectively. It is critical to speak with a veterinarian to identify the appropriate dietary changes and ensure that the dog's nutritional demands are addressed while also supporting their individual health needs.

How to adjust your dog's diet based on their activity level

When selecting dog food for dogs with special health concerns, it is critical to avoid common errors to ensure that the chosen diet properly satisfies their individual demands. Here are some pointers to help you avoid these pitfalls:

1. Consult a veterinarian before making any dietary changes: Before making any dietary adjustments, it is critical to consult with a veterinarian who can provide advise based on the dog's individual health situation. They can advise on the best diet for you and assist you avoid any potential allergens or substances.

2. Read the ingredient labels of dog food carefully to detect potential allergens or ingredients that may not be suited for dogs with specific health conditions. Look for low-allergen or hypoallergenic meals that omit common allergies including wheat, maize, soy, and certain proteins like chicken or beef.

3. Avoid unneeded additives: Some dog diets may contain unnecessary additives, preservatives, or artificial components that may aggravate a dog's health. Choose dog foods with natural and high-quality ingredients over ones with a lot of fillers or artificial additives.

4. Consider the nutrient profile: Ensure that the dog food you choose contains the nutrients your dog requires for his or her specific health condition. Diets for dogs with renal disease, for example, should be low in phosphorus and high

in high-quality protein, whereas diets for dogs with joint difficulties should include substances that promote joint health, such as glucosamine and omega-3 fatty acids.

5. After moving to a new food, regularly observe the dog's response as well as any changes in their health state. If the problem does not improve or worsens, consult a veterinarian to examine the food and make any required changes.

6. Avoid overfeeding: To avoid overfeeding, carefully measure and monitor the portions of dog food, especially for dogs with obesity or weight management concerns. To establish the right amount size for the dog's unique needs, follow the manufacturer's feeding guidelines or contact with a veterinarian.

7. Consider the dog's preferences: While it is critical to select a diet that suits the dog's unique health needs, it is also crucial to consider the dog's preferences and taste. If your dog refuses to eat the prescribed diet, talk to your veterinarian about additional options or ways to make the food more enticing.

Dog owners may choose the best diet for their dog's general health and well-being by avoiding these frequent errors and taking into account the dog's individual health condition, nutritional needs, and preferences. Regular monitoring and consultation with a veterinarian are required to verify that the chosen food continues to adequately satisfy the demands of the dog.

Chapter 5: The Role of Supplements in Your Dog's Diet

It is critical to evaluate all aspects of a dog's diet, including the effect of supplements, when selecting the correct dog food for dogs with certain health concerns. Supplements can be quite beneficial in meeting a dog's individual demands and addressing certain health concerns. However, it is critical to understand how to use supplements correctly and avoid frequent problems.

Supplements can provide extra nutrients or therapeutic benefits that a dog's usual diet may lack. They can benefit joint health, digestion, the immune system, and a variety of other health conditions. However, before putting any supplements into a dog's food, speak with a veterinarian. A veterinarian can evaluate the dog's individual health condition and propose supplements to augment their dietary needs.

Reading and comprehending supplement ingredient labels is just as important as reading dog food labels. It is critical to select high-quality supplements that are free of needless additions, fillers, or artificial substances that could aggravate a dog's health. Monitoring the dog's reaction to the supplements is also necessary to ensure their effectiveness.

In this chapter, we will look at the importance of supplements in a dog's diet when it comes to treating particular health issues. We'll go over typical traps to avoid, factors to consider when selecting supplements, and how to track their effectiveness. Dog owners may provide the greatest possible support for their furry companions' unique health needs by knowing the significance of supplements and making informed decisions.

The benefits of supplements for dogs

Supplements can give several benefits for pets suffering from specific medical ailments. They can assist in addressing deficits in their usual diet as well as providing additional support to boost their general well-being. Here are some of the most important advantages of dog supplements:

1. Nutritional Support: Dogs with specific health issues may have nutritional requirements that are not supplied by ordinary dog food alone. Supplements can help people with certain health issues by providing extra vitamins, minerals, and other critical nutrients. Dogs with joint problems, for example, may benefit from supplements containing glucosamine and chondroitin, which support joint health and reduce inflammation.

2. Joint Supplements: Many dogs, especially those who are elderly or have arthritis, can benefit from joint supplements. These supplements frequently include substances such as glucosamine, chondroitin, and omega-3 fatty acids, which can help reduce joint pain and inflammation, increase mobility, and promote cartilage health.

3. Digestive Health: Supplements that support digestive health can help dogs who have digestive concerns such as food allergies or gastrointestinal diseases. Probiotics, for example, can aid in the restoration of healthy bacteria in the stomach, improve digestion, and ease symptoms such as diarrhea or constipation.

4. Immune System Support: Antioxidants, vitamins, and minerals in supplements can help improve a dog's immune system and protect him from common ailments. These supplements can help to boost the body's natural defense mechanisms while also promoting overall health and vigor.

5. Skin and Coat Health: Supplements that promote healthy skin and a lustrous coat may aid dogs with skin allergies or dull coats. Omega-3 fatty acids, such as those found in fish oil supplements, can help reduce inflammation, relieve itching, and enhance skin and coat quality.

6. Cognitive Function: Supplements that enhance brain health and cognitive function may aid older canines or those with cognitive impairment. Antioxidants, omega-3 fatty acids, and vitamins B6 and B12 can all assist to boost memory, focus, and overall mental health.

While supplements can bring considerable benefits, they should not be used in place of a well-balanced and healthy diet. They should be used as a supplement to a dog's regular diet and under the supervision of a veterinarian. Regular monitoring of the dog's response to the supplements is essential to verify their effectiveness and, if necessary, change the dosage.

Finally, vitamins can be extremely beneficial in helping dogs with specific health issues. They can supplement nutrients, correct deficiencies, and improve many areas of a dog's health. To ensure the best possible support for a dog's individual health needs, it is critical to consult with a veterinarian, purchase high-quality supplements, and evaluate their performance.

Common supplements and their uses

There are various supplements that are commonly used to treat certain health issues in dogs. These supplements can provide focused assistance and help dogs' general health. Here are a couple such examples:

1. Glucosamine and Chondroitin: These supplements are often used to maintain joint health in dogs, particularly those suffering from arthritis or other joint problems. Glucosamine supports cartilage integrity, and chondroitin promotes cartilage healing. These vitamins can help with

joint pain and inflammation, as well as mobility and overall joint health.

2. Omega-3 Fatty Acids: Omega-3 fatty acids, such as those found in fish oil supplements, can help dogs with a number of health issues. They offer anti-inflammatory characteristics that can aid in the relief of joint discomfort, the improvement of skin and coat health, and the enhancement of cognitive function. Omega-3 fatty acids can help enhance the immune system and improve cardiovascular health.

3. Probiotics: Probiotic pills contain healthy bacteria that can assist dogs with digestive difficulties restore the balance of gut flora. They can help with digestion, relieve symptoms such as diarrhea and constipation, and maintain a healthy gut environment. Probiotics can be especially beneficial for dogs that have dietary allergies, gastrointestinal issues, or are on antibiotics.

4. Antioxidants, such as vitamins C and E, can help enhance a dog's immune system and protect against oxidative stress caused by free radicals. They can improve general health and energy while also lowering the risk of

chronic diseases. Antioxidants are also anti-inflammatory, which can help dogs with joint problems or skin allergies.

5. Vitamin and mineral supplements: Vitamin and mineral supplements may aid dogs who have specific dietary deficiencies. Dogs with a vitamin D deficit, for example, may benefit from supplementation to promote bone health. Dogs with low iron levels may also require iron supplements to avoid anemia. It is critical to speak with a veterinarian to evaluate a dog's individual dietary needs and to select the appropriate supplements.

6. Herbal supplements, such as turmeric or milk thistle, are used to promote numerous areas of a dog's health. Turmeric has anti-inflammatory effects that can help dogs who have joint problems or allergies. Milk thistle is frequently used to aid in liver function and cleansing.

To ensure their effectiveness and safety, it is critical to select high-quality supplements from trustworthy producers. It is also critical to adhere to the suggested dosage and monitor the dog's reaction to the supplements. Regular contact with a veterinarian is required to monitor the dog's progress, modify the dosage as needed, and ensure that the supplements are producing the intended results.

In conclusion, popular dog vitamins can provide focused support for various health concerns. Glucosamine and chondroitin promote joint health, omega-3 fatty acids increase overall well-being, probiotics aid digestion, antioxidants strengthen the immune system, vitamin and mineral supplements address nutritional shortages, and herbal supplements provide a variety of health advantages. To ensure the best possible support for a dog's individual health needs, it is critical to consult with a veterinarian, purchase high-quality supplements, and evaluate their performance.

How to choose the right supplements for your dog

There are various variables to consider while selecting the proper vitamins for your dog to ensure their effectiveness and safety. Here are some pointers to help you make an educated decision:

1. Consult a Veterinarian: Before beginning any supplements for your dog, you must first consult with a veterinarian. They may evaluate your dog's individual health requirements, offer appropriate supplements, and advise you on dosage and length of use. A veterinarian will have a thorough overview of your dog's medical history and will be able to provide knowledgeable recommendations based on their knowledge.

2. Investigate reputed Manufacturers: It is critical to select supplements from reputed manufacturers who adhere to high quality control standards. Look for organizations with a strong reputation, high-quality ingredients, and third-party testing to assure product purity and potency. Reading customer reviews and seeking suggestions from reputable sources can also assist you in locating trustworthy supplement brands.

3. Read the components List: Before purchasing any supplement for your dog, carefully read the components list. Check that the active ingredients are listed correctly and that there are no extraneous fillers or additions. Supplements with artificial colors, flavors, or preservatives

should be avoided. When feasible, choose natural and organic products.

4. Consider Your Dog's special Needs: Every dog is different, and their special health needs should be considered while selecting supplements. Consider aspects such as your dog's age, breed, size, and any current health conditions. For example, if your dog has joint problems, glucosamine and chondroitin supplements may be therapeutic. Probiotic supplements may be beneficial if your dog has stomach difficulties.

5. Examine the Dosage and Form: Check the supplement's recommended dosage and make sure it's acceptable for your dog's size and weight. Some supplements are available in tablet, pill, powder, or liquid form. When selecting a supplement form, keep your dog's preferences and simplicity of administration in mind. Some dogs may prefer chewable tablets, but others may prefer liquids combined with their chow.

6. Monitor Your Dog's Response: Once you've decided on a supplement and begun giving it to your dog, keep a close eye on how they react. Examine their health state for any

evidence of improvement or any harmful reactions. If you detect any side effects or no improvement, call your veterinarian to re-evaluate the supplement's suitability or dosage.

7. Follow Recommended Guidelines: Always follow the manufacturer's and your veterinarian's recommended guidelines. Excessive supplementation can be hazardous to your dog's health. To get the greatest benefits, stick to the suggested dosage and period of use.

Finally, selecting the correct supplements for your dog entails speaking with a veterinarian, investigating trustworthy manufacturers, reading ingredient lists, taking into account your dog's individual needs, analysing dosage and form, monitoring your dog's response, and adhering to prescribed standards. You can make an informed decision and provide focused support to improve your dog's overall well-being if you consider these issues.

Chapter 6: Creating a Feeding Schedule for Your Dog

Developing a feeding regimen for your dog is critical to their general health and well-being. Dogs, like humans, require a well-balanced and steady diet in order to flourish. However, choosing the proper feeding schedule can be difficult because it is dependent on a variety of characteristics such as age, breed, size, activity level, and dietary demands. You may develop a feeding schedule that ensures your dog gets the right quantity of nutrition at the right times by following simple rules.

First, consult with your veterinarian to evaluate your dog's exact dietary needs. They can advise you on the type of food, portion quantities, and frequency of feeding based on your dog's specific requirements. Age, weight, and any current health conditions will all play a role in choosing the best feeding plan.
Next, select a high-quality dog food that matches renowned organizations' nutritional requirements. Check the ingredient list to be sure it contains vital elements including

protein, carbs, healthy fats, vitamins, and minerals. Foods containing artificial additions or fillers should be avoided.

Once you've chosen the appropriate cuisine, divide the daily recommended portion into two or three meals throughout the day. Puppies and younger dogs may require more frequent feedings, although mature dogs can often be fed twice daily. Set precise feeding times for your dog and keep to them consistently to build a pattern.

Finally, keep a close eye on your dog's weight and overall health. To maintain a healthy weight, adjust portion amounts and feeding frequency as needed. Always supply fresh water and minimize overfeeding or free-feeding, which can lead to obesity and other health problems.

You can ensure that your dog obtains sufficient nourishment and maintains maximum health by designing a feeding schedule tailored to his or her unique needs and following these instructions.

The importance of a consistent feeding schedule

A consistent feeding plan is critical for the overall health and well-being of a dog. Dogs, like people, rely on regularity and structure, and sticking to a feeding plan allows them to build a sense of security and predictability in their daily life. A constant feeding schedule is vital for the following reasons:

1. Dogs' digestive systems are sensitive, and rapid changes in their food schedule might disturb their digestive process. Consistency allows their bodies to acclimate and regulate digestion, lowering the likelihood of gastrointestinal disorders like diarrhea, constipation, or upset stomach.

2. Energy Levels: Maintaining a consistent feeding plan ensures that your dog gets the right quantity of nutrition at the right times. This keeps their energy levels up throughout the day and gives them the food they need for physical activities and exercise.

3. Weight Control: Consistency in feeding times and quantity quantities is critical in controlling your dog's weight. You may limit the amount of food your dog

consumes by following a consistent feeding schedule, preventing overeating or underfeeding. This is especially crucial in the prevention of obesity, which can lead to a variety of health issues such as joint pain, heart disease, and diabetes.

4. Training and Behavior: A regular feeding plan can also aid with training and behavior control. Routine is important to dogs, and having established feeding times can help you establish other training routines, such as toilet training or obedience training. A consistent eating schedule can also help reduce behavioral concerns like food anger or begging.

5. Feeding time is an excellent moment for bonding and developing a strong relationship with your dog. You may reinforce trust and create a pleasant link with food by continuously being present throughout meal times. This can also assist to reduce resource guarding and foster a good bond between you and your dog.

Finally, a regular feeding schedule is critical for your dog's overall health, digestion, weight management, training, temperament, and relationship with you. By developing and sticking to a regimen, you can guarantee that your furry friend receives proper nutrition, maintains maximum health, and lives a happy and rewarding life.

Tips for establishing a feeding routine

Creating a feeding regimen for your dog is not only good for their health and well-being, but it also helps them feel more structured and stable in their daily lives. Here are some pointers to help you develop a regular feeding schedule:

1. Determine the Appropriate Portion Size: Talk to your veterinarian about the best portion size for your dog based on their age, breed, size, and activity level. This will guarantee that kids get the proper quantity of nutrition without overeating or undereating.

2. Fix Meal Times: Set specific meal times for your dog and adhere to them consistently. Dogs should ideally be fed two to three times per day, depending on their age and dietary requirements. Create a plan that works for you and your dog's routine, allowing adequate time between meals for digesting.

3. Avoid Free Feeding: Free feeding, which involves leaving food available for your dog to graze on all day, can contribute to overeating and weight gain. To avoid overconsumption, schedule meal times and eliminate any uneaten food after a specified length of time.

4. Measuring Cups: To correctly measure your dog's food servings, use measuring cups or a kitchen scale. This will assist to prevent overfeeding and ensure that they receive the proper amount of nutrients.

5. Maintain the Same Food Brand and Type: Sudden changes in your dog's diet can cause stomach distress. Unless otherwise directed by your veterinarian, stick to the same brand and type of food. If you must change their food, do so gradually over several days by mixing small portions of the new food with the old.

6. Make a Feeding Area: Choose a location in your home where your dog will be fed. This will help them develop a routine and keep them from begging or scavenging for food in other parts of the house.

7. Make It a Point to Be Present throughout Meal Times: Make it a point to be present throughout your dog's meal times. This will help to build trust and a favorable relationship with food. It also allows you to keep track of their eating habits and ensure they are eating correctly.

8. Avoid Feeding Table Scraps: It is advised to avoid giving your dog table scraps or human food as treats. Human food can be harmful to dogs' health and interrupt their balanced diet. Stick to high-quality dog treats or check your veterinarian for acceptable substitutes.

9. Be Consistent: Establishing a feeding habit requires consistency. Maintain the same routine and portion amounts every day, including on weekends and holidays. Dogs thrive on regularity, and constancy makes them feel safe and secure.

You can assure your dog's best health, digestion, weight management, training, behavior, and a strong link with you by following these suggestions and maintaining a consistent feeding regimen. Remember to seek specialized guidance from your veterinarian based on your dog's individual needs.

How to monitor your dog's weight and adjust their feeding schedule as needed

Maintaining your dog's overall health and well-being requires you to monitor their weight and change their food regimen as appropriate. Here are some tips to help you effectively monitor your dog's weight and make appropriate food adjustments:

1. Regular Weigh-Ins: Begin by weighing your dog on a regular basis to note any weight changes. This can be done at home with a scale or at your veterinarian's office. Weighing them once a month is usually fine, but if your dog is overweight or has certain health concerns, more frequent weigh-ins may be required.

2. Assess Body Condition: In addition to weighing your dog, you should evaluate their overall health. This entails visually and physically inspecting their body to determine whether they are underweight, overweight, or at their target weight. Examine your ribs, waistline, and overall muscular tone for apparent indicators. Your veterinarian can advise

you on what constitutes a healthy body condition for your individual dog breed.

3. Consult Your Veterinarian: If you detect any substantial changes in your dog's weight or body condition, you should consult your veterinarian. They may offer professional advice and help on how to change your dog's feeding schedule and portion amounts based on their individual needs.

4. meal Control: If your dog is gaining weight, you may need to lower their meal portions. However, if they are losing weight or are underweight, they may need to increase their portion sizes. Your veterinarian can advise you on the best changes to make based on your dog's age, breed, size, and activity level.

5. Feeding demeanour: Keep an eye on your dog's eating habits and demeanour throughout meal times. If kids routinely leave food on the plate or appear hungry soon after eating, it could be an indication that their portion sizes need to be adjusted. Similarly, if they finish their meals quickly and clamour for more, it could be an indication that their portion sizes are too large.

6. Consider Treats and Snacks: When tracking your dog's weight, you should also consider the treats and snacks he or she receives throughout the day. These extra calories can lead to weight gain. Limiting the amount and size of treats or choosing low-calorie alternatives will help you efficiently manage your dog's weight.

7. Frequent Exercise: In addition to changing their meal plan, frequent exercise is critical for your dog's weight and overall health. Consult your veterinarian to decide the best exercise plan for your dog based on its age, breed, and physical condition.

You can ensure that your dog maintains a healthy weight and enjoys optimal health and well-being by periodically monitoring their weight, examining their bodily condition, consulting with your veterinarian, and making appropriate adjustments to their food schedule and portion sizes. Always seek professional counsel from your veterinarian for tailored advice based on your dog's individual needs.

Chapter 7: Addressing Common Nutritional Concerns for Dogs

Proper diet is essential for a dog's general health and well-being. Monitoring your pet's weight and making any adjustments to their feeding plan is an important part of ensuring that they get the proper nourishment. You may help avoid obesity, which can contribute to a variety of health issues in dogs, by doing so.

In this article, we will go over how to accurately monitor your dog's weight and make necessary adjustments to their feeding plan. We will discuss the significance of regular weigh-ins, checking body condition, talking with your veterinarian, changing portion sizes, monitoring feeding behavior, introducing treats and snacks, and incorporating regular exercise into your dog's routine.

By following these steps and consulting with your veterinarian, you may address common nutritional difficulties for dogs and ensure that your canine companion maintains a healthy weight and enjoys optimal health. This guide will provide you with the information you need to make informed decisions regarding your dog's diet, whether you need to assist your dog lose a few pounds or ensure they are getting enough nutrition to maintain a healthy weight.

Remember that each dog is unique, and their nutritional requirements may differ depending on factors such as age, breed, size, and activity level. It is always better to seek personalized advice from your veterinarian regarding your dog's specific needs.

Allergies and intolerances

Allergies and intolerances can also impact a dog's overall health and well-being, particularly when it comes to nutrition. Dogs, like people, can acquire food allergies or intolerances to specific foods or ingredients. These diseases can have a major impact on their weight and general health.

Canine allergies are immunological responses to certain proteins in food. Beef, chicken, dairy, wheat, and soy are common food allergies in dogs. When a dog consumes certain allergens, his or her immune system reacts, causing symptoms such as itching, skin rashes, gastrointestinal discomfort, and even respiratory problems. Allergies can also cause weight loss or trouble gaining weight if the dog avoids eating because it is uncomfortable.

Intolerances, on the other hand, are not the same as allergies. They are caused by a dog's digestive tract having difficulties breaking down particular components in food and do not involve the immune system. Lactose intolerance, for example, is frequent in dogs because they lack the enzyme lactase, which is required to digest lactose, the sugar present in milk and dairy products. This might cause stomach discomfort, such as diarrhea or vomiting.

Allergies and intolerances must be considered while monitoring a dog's weight and making adjustments to their feeding regimen. If your dog has been diagnosed with a food allergy or intolerance, you must avoid giving them any meals or treats that include the allergen or substance to which they are sensitive.

In these circumstances, consulting with your veterinarian is critical because they can help identify the exact allergen or intolerance through diagnostic tests or elimination diets. They can then propose suitable replacement meals or advise on how to manage the disease through dietary changes.

When purchasing commercial dog food or treats, it is equally critical to carefully study the labels and ingredient lists. Look for items designed expressly for dogs with allergies or intolerances, or provide a hypoallergenic or limited ingredient diet.

Finally, allergies and intolerances can have a large impact on a dog's weight and overall health. When modifying a dog's feeding schedule and monitoring their weight, it is critical to consider any known allergies or intolerances and make appropriate nutritional adjustments. Consultation with a veterinarian is essential for properly recognizing and controlling these issues, as well as ensuring that your pet obtains the nourishment they require to maintain a healthy weight and overall health.

Weight management

Weight control is critical to a dog's overall health and well-being, especially when allergies and intolerances are present. Due to a variety of circumstances, allergies and intolerances can contribute to weight loss or trouble gaining weight in dogs.

For starters, allergies in dogs can cause weight loss. When a dog is allergic to specific foods or components, they may develop itching, skin rashes, or gastrointestinal problems. This might lead to weight loss by reducing appetite or avoiding particular foods. Furthermore, if the dog's immune system is constantly active as a result of allergies, it can produce chronic inflammation, affecting their metabolism and preventing weight gain.

In contrast, intolerances can have an impact on a dog's weight management. Lactose intolerance, for example, is widespread in dogs, and consuming dairy products can cause digestive problems, including diarrhea or vomiting. These symptoms can result in weight reduction by causing a decrease in appetite or avoidance of meals. Furthermore, if a dog's digestive tract is unable to adequately break down specific compounds in food, it might impact vitamin absorption and utilization, potentially resulting in nutrient shortages and weight loss.

It is critical to identify and avoid certain allergens or intolerant components when it comes to regulating a dog's weight in connection to allergies and intolerances. A veterinarian is essential in this procedure because they can run diagnostic testing or propose elimination diets to determine the exact allergen or intolerance. Once the problematic elements have been identified, appropriate dietary alterations can be made to exclude them from the dog's diet.

It is critical to choose commercial dog food or treats that are specifically made for dogs with allergies or intolerances when it comes to weight management. To reduce the danger of provoking allergic responses or digestive difficulties, these goods are frequently created with alternate protein sources or limited ingredient lists. Hypoallergenic or limited ingredient diets can also be explored for dogs with allergies or intolerances because they provide a controlled and easily digestible food alternative.

Regularly monitoring a dog's weight is critical for general health management. If a dog is losing weight or having trouble gaining weight due to allergies or intolerances, it is critical to check with a veterinarian to ensure proper nutritional changes are addressed. They may advise on feeding schedules and amount sizes, as well as offer suitable replacement foods that match the nutritional needs of the dog while eliminating allergies or intolerant substances.

Finally, weight management is important for a dog's overall health, especially when allergies and intolerances are prevalent. Weight loss or trouble gaining weight can result from allergies, whereas intolerances can impact nutritional absorption and utilization, potentially leading to weight loss. Identifying and avoiding allergens or intolerant substances through suitable dietary changes is critical in efficiently regulating a dog's weight. Consultation with a veterinarian and the selection of appropriate commercial dog food or treats intended for dogs with allergies or intolerances are critical stages in maintaining a healthy weight and optimal health in dogs with these issues.

Dental health and nutrition

Dental health and nutrition in dogs are intimately tied to weight control and overall health, particularly when allergies and intolerances are present. Poor oral health can impair a dog's ability to effectively eat and chew, resulting in weight loss or difficulties gaining weight. Furthermore, the quality of nutrients and the type of food a dog consumes can have an effect on their oral health.

For starters, dental problems such as tooth decay, gum disease, or tooth loss can make eating painful or uncomfortable for a dog. This might lead to weight loss by reducing appetite or avoiding particular foods. Dogs who have dental issues may have difficulties digesting their food, which can contribute to weight loss since they are unable to swallow their meals adequately.

Furthermore, poor tooth health might impair nutritional digestion and absorption. When a dog has dental problems, they may be unable to effectively break down their food, resulting in decreased nutrient absorption. Even if the dog consumes an adequate amount of food, this can result in vitamin shortages and hamper weight increase. As a result, maintaining good tooth health is essential for healthy digestion and nutrient utilization.

In terms of nutrition, the sort of food a dog eats can have an effect on their oral health. Maintaining healthy teeth and gums requires feeding a balanced and nutritious food that satisfies the dog's individual nutritional demands. Commercial dog diets of high quality are formulated to supply the nutrients required for overall health, including dental health. These foods frequently contain components that enhance dental hygiene, such as crunchy kibble, which aids in the cleaning of teeth and the reduction of plaque formation.

Furthermore, certain foods can contribute to tooth problems in dogs. Feeding dogs, a diet strong in carbs or sugars, for example, can raise the risk of teeth decay and gum disease. These chemicals can adhere to the teeth and serve as a breeding environment for germs, resulting in dental issues. Choosing dental-friendly nibbles or chews over sugary treats or table scraps will help promote healthy dental health.

Regular dental treatment is also essential for a dog's dental health. Brushing their teeth on a regular basis with a dog-friendly toothpaste, providing dental chews or toys that assist clean teeth, and arranging frequent dental check-ups with a veterinarian are all part of this. These practices can aid in the prevention of dental disorders as well as the early discovery and treatment of any concerns that do emerge.

Finally, oral health and nutrition are inextricably linked to weight control and overall health in dogs, especially when allergies and intolerances are present. Weight loss or difficulties gaining weight might be exacerbated by poor dental health due to pain or discomfort while eating. Furthermore, the type of food a dog consumes can have an impact on their dental health, and giving a balanced and nutritious diet is critical for maintaining good teeth and gums. Brushing, administering dental chews, and scheduling check-ups are all important habits in promoting good dental health. Dog owners may safeguard their pets' general well-being and optimal health by addressing dental health and nutrition alongside weight management.

Chapter 8: The Impact of Nutrition on Your Dog's Health and Longevity

Good nutrition is critical to the general health and lifespan of our canine companions. Dental health and nutrition are intimately related to weight control and overall well-being in dogs, especially in cases involving allergies and intolerances. Poor oral health can impair a dog's ability to effectively eat and chew, resulting in weight loss or difficulties gaining weight. Furthermore, the quality of nutrients and the type of food a dog consumes can have an effect on their oral health. Tooth decay, gum disease, or tooth loss can make eating difficult for a dog, resulting in a diminished appetite or avoidance of particular meals. Furthermore, poor tooth health can impair food digestion and absorption, resulting in dietary deficits and a lack of weight gain. It is critical to feed a balanced and nutritious diet that fulfils a dog's individual nutritional demands in order to maintain healthy teeth and gums. Dental hygiene is promoted by high-quality commercial dog diets, and avoiding sugary snacks or table scraps can help prevent dental problems. Brushing, administering dental chews, and scheduling check-ups are also important in promoting good dental health. Dog owners may safeguard their pets' general well-being and optimal health for years to come by addressing dental health and nutrition with weight management.

How proper nutrition can prevent common health issues in dogs

Proper nutrition is critical in preventing common health issues in dogs, including dental health and weight management. Dog owners can help prevent different dental diseases and maintain their furry companions' overall well-being by offering a balanced and healthy diet.

Periodontal disease, caused by plaque and tartar build-up on the teeth, is one of the most prevalent dental disorders in dogs. Gum inflammation, dental damage, and even tooth loss can result from this illness. Feeding a high-quality commercial dog food designed expressly to encourage oral hygiene can help minimize plaque and tartar build-up. These foods frequently feature a crunchy texture that helps to mechanically clean the dog's teeth while he chews, lowering the risk of dental disease.

Furthermore, appropriate nutrition can help dogs avoid weight-related health problems. Obesity is a big concern in pets, and it can lead to a variety of health conditions such as diabetes, heart disease, and joint difficulties. Overweight or obese dogs are more likely to have dental problems due to increased pressure on their teeth and gums. Dog owners can assist their canines maintain a healthy weight and reduce the risk of dental disorders by offering a balanced and portion-controlled food.

When dogs have allergies or intolerances, correct nutrition is even more important. Allergies can cause skin discomfort, gastrointestinal disorders, and even tooth problems. Dog owners can prevent allergy reactions that may impact their pet's oral health by identifying and eliminating allergens from their dog's diet, such as specific proteins or grains. Furthermore, eating a diet designed specifically for dogs with allergies can help ease symptoms and boost overall oral health.

Furthermore, adequate feeding ensures that dogs get all of the nutrients they need for good health. Nutrient shortages can weaken the immune system and make dogs more vulnerable to a variety of health concerns, including dental disorders. Owners may strengthen their pets' immune systems and encourage healthy teeth and gums by giving a balanced and complete food that covers all of their nutritional needs.

Finally, good nutrition is critical in preventing common health issues in dogs, notably dental health and weight control. A balanced and nutritious diet that fulfils a dog's individual nutritional demands can aid in the prevention of dental issues such as periodontal disease and tooth decay. Furthermore, keeping a healthy weight through good eating might lower the risk of dental disorders and other weight-related health concerns. Dog owners may safeguard their pets' entire well-being and encourage optimal health for years to come by addressing oral health and nutrition together.

The role of nutrition in promoting a long and healthy life for your dog

Proper nutrition is critical for supporting a long and healthy life for dogs, particularly in terms of dental health and weight management. Dog owners may prevent common health disorders and ensure their furry pets enjoy a happy and active life by offering a balanced and nutritious diet.

Firstly, nutrition plays a key part in maintaining excellent oral health in dogs. Periodontal disease is one of the most prevalent dental problems in dogs, and if left untreated, it can lead to major difficulties. Feeding a high-quality commercial dog food that encourages dental care will help prevent plaque and tartar formation on the teeth. These diets are frequently made with special components that assist mechanically clean the dog's teeth while he chews, lowering the risk of dental disease. Dogs can avoid pain, discomfort, and potential tooth loss by preventing dental disorders, resulting in a longer and healthier life.

Second, correct nourishment is essential for dog weight management. Obesity is a major issue in pets, and it can have serious ramifications for their general health. Overweight or obese dogs are at a higher risk of having a variety of health problems, including diabetes, heart disease, and joint difficulties. Dog owners can assist their canines maintain a healthy weight and lower the risk of dental problems linked with obesity by giving a balanced and portion-controlled food. Maintaining a healthy weight enhances mobility and energy levels, helping dogs to live an active and satisfying life.

Furthermore, for dogs with allergies or intolerances, correct nutrition is critical. Allergies can cause a variety of difficulties in dogs, including dental problems. Dog owners can prevent allergy reactions that may affect their pet's oral health by identifying and eliminating allergens from their dog's diet, such as specific proteins or grains. Feeding a meal designed specifically for dogs with allergies can help relieve symptoms and improve overall oral health. Dogs can enjoy a comfortable and healthy life without the issues associated with allergy reactions if allergies are addressed through adequate feeding.

Finally, offering a balanced and complete food ensures that dogs obtain all of the nutrients they require for optimal health. Nutrient shortages can weaken the immune system and make dogs more vulnerable to a variety of health concerns, including dental disorders. Owners may boost their pets' immune systems and maintain healthy teeth and gums by satisfying all of their nutritional needs for dogs through adequate diet. As a result, dogs live longer and better lives.

Finally, diet is critical in fostering a long and healthy life for dogs. Dog owners can prevent common health issues such as dental problems and obesity by giving a balanced and healthy food. Proper nutrition also treats allergies and ensures that dogs receive all of the nutrients they require for maximum health. Dog owners may ensure their pet companions live happy and active lives for years to come by addressing nutrition.

Conclusion

Finally, when it comes to dog nutrition, the adage "you are what you eat" is true. A balanced and nutritious diet is critical for supporting optimal health and lifespan in our four-legged friends. Dog owners may ensure that their canines enjoy a happy and active life by focusing on dental health, weight control, allergies, and total nutrient consumption.

Dental health is an important element of a dog's overall wellness. We can avoid plaque and tartar build-up and reduce the risk of periodontal disease by feeding high-quality commercial dog food that encourages oral hygiene. This not only relieves our dogs' pain and discomfort, but it also helps them keep their sparkling whites for many years to come.

Another important component in fostering a long and healthy life for our dogs is weight management. We can prevent obesity and its accompanying health problems, such as diabetes and joint difficulties, by providing a balanced and portion-controlled diet. Maintaining a healthy weight for our four-legged pals helps them to have an active lifestyle and ensures their general well-being.

It is also critical to address allergies with good nutrition. We can prevent allergic reactions in our dogs' dental health by identifying and eliminating allergens from their food. Feeding them a food designed specifically for dogs with allergies not only relieves symptoms but also improves overall oral health.

Finally, it is critical for our dogs' immune systems and overall health to ensure that they obtain all of the necessary nutrients through correct feeding. Nutrient shortages can weaken their immune systems, making them more vulnerable to a variety of health problems. We can boost their immune system, maintain good teeth and gums, and eventually lengthen their longevity by satisfying their dietary needs.

Finally, by emphasizing dog nutrition, we can lay the groundwork for our canine companions to live a long and healthy life. A balanced and nutritious diet is the key to achieving optimal health and longevity for our beloved dogs, from dental health to weight control, allergies, and overall nutritional consumption. So let's feed them well and watch them grow!

Final Note

Congratulations on seeing the end of this book!

I want to use this medium to thank you for your purchase and reading. And I do hope that this book serves as a guide to understanding and providing the needed care for your canine friend to live a healthy life.

If this book has given an insight on how to care for your trusted friend, please you will do well to leave a positive feedback and recommend it to others who can equally find it useful in taking proper nutritional are of their canine friend. Your insights can help others in providing the needed nutritional needs in ensuring their overall well-being and quality of life.

Thanks again and I wish you and your best friend a long friendly and healthy life.